AROMATHERAPY FOR BEGINNERS

Essential Oils, Healing Blends, And Natural Wellness Techniques For Stress Relief, Better Sleep, And Enhanced Mood

DR SAWYER DIEGO

Copyright © [2024] by [Dr. .Sawyer Diego]. All rights reserved.

Except for brief quotations included in critical reviews and certain other noncommercial uses allowed by copyright law, no part of this publication may be reproduced, distributed, or transmitted in any form or by any means, including photocopying, recording, or other electronic or mechanical methods, without the publisher's prior written permission.

DISCLAMER

Nothing in this book should be interpreted as medical advice; it is meant exclusively for educational reasons. Regarding their specific health issues and treatment options, readers are urged to speak with licensed healthcare professionals. The publisher and author disclaim all liability for any errors or omissions in the material provided, as well as for any negative effects that may arise from using or abusing the information. Although every attempt has been taken to guarantee that the material in this book is correct as of the date of publishing, new research may have superseded some of the content because medical knowledge is always changing. It is recommended that readers confirm the most recent medical recommendations and guidelines. The reader of this book undertakes to release the author and publisher from any claims or liabilities resulting from the use of this information, and understands and accepts the inherent risks connected with healthcare decisions.

TABLE OF CONTENTS

ABOUT THE BOOK

Aromatherapy for Beginners" is a must-have resource for anyone interested in the therapeutic potential of essential oils. It explores the origins and rich history of aromatherapy, tracing its origins and examining fundamental principles that underpin its efficacy.

It also sheds light on the wide variety of available essential oils, outlining their distinct qualities and the various extraction techniques. In addition to their pleasant scents, readers learn how these oils can benefit emotional well-being, reduce stress, and even boost immunity.

Whether you're looking to enhance relaxation at home, incorporate oils into skincare routines, or explore their role in emotional support, this book's practical approach will help beginners integrate aromatherapy seamlessly into their daily lives. It offers comprehensive insights into creating an ideal aromatherapy space, essential tools required for safe usage and crucial safety precautions to ensure a positive experience. Each technique is carefully explained with step-by-step guidance.

Readers will find specialized chapters devoted to addressing specific needs like anxiety, headaches, digestive health, and respiratory issues through tailored aromatherapeutic practices; for those eager to craft their blends, a collection of do-it-yourself recipes offers practical instructions for creating everything from soothing bath salts to invigorating massage oils and refreshing room sprays. The health and wellness benefits of aromatherapy are extensively covered, from reducing anxiety and managing pain to improving sleep quality and boosting overall immunity.

Aromatherapy can be incorporated into a variety of contexts, such as offices, yoga classes, and even travel situations. Safety is emphasized at all times, with thorough instructions on how to dilute essential oils, deal with sensitivity issues, and take into account particular populations, such as expectant mothers or people on medication.

Frequently asked questions are answered openly and honestly, debunking myths and offering trustworthy resources to assist in making educated decisions.

"Aromatherapy for Beginners" is more than just a book; it's a doorway to learning about the life-changing potential of essential oils. It gives readers the skills and assurance they need to successfully utilize aromatherapy's healing properties, which enhance mental and physical health.

CHAPTER ONE
AROMATHERAPY OVERVIEW
AROMATHERAPY: WHAT IS IT?

Aromatherapy is a holistic healing modality that uses naturally occurring plant extracts, or essential oils, to support mental, emotional, and physical well-being. These aromatic oils are extracted from different plant parts, such as flowers, leaves, roots, and bark, using methods like steam distillation or cold pressing.

Each essential oil has a unique aroma and therapeutic qualities that can affect mood, reduce stress, improve relaxation, and even support physical healing. Aromatherapists believe that essential oils interact with the limbic system of the body, which is in charge of emotions and memories, causing responses that can facilitate healing or promote relaxation.

For example, lavender oil is well-known for its calming properties, which make it perfect for lowering anxiety and enhancing the quality of sleep.

On the other hand, peppermint oil is well-known for its invigorating properties, which are often used to boost energy levels and relieve headaches.

Because essential oils are so versatile, people can customize their aromatherapy practices to meet a variety of needs, such as enhancing focus during work or creating a calming environment for relaxation at home.

ADVANTAGES OF AROMATHERAPY

Aromatherapy has many advantages in the physical, emotional, and psychological domains, which is why it is a widely used and adaptable modality across the globe. In the physical domain, essential oils can support conditions like respiratory disorders, muscle aches, and skin irritations. In the emotional and mental domains, aromatherapy encourages relaxation and stress relief, which can improve mood and mental clarity. For example, inhaling citrus oils like lemon or orange can uplift mood and reduce feelings of depression.

In complementary medicine, aromatherapy is also used to support conventional treatments and helps manage chronic conditions such as insomnia, anxiety disorders, and nausea. Because of its non-invasive nature and low side effects, aromatherapy is a preferred option for people looking for natural alternatives to pharmaceutical interventions. Aromatherapy practices are also easy to incorporate into daily routines, such as diffusing essential oils in the home, adding them to bathwater, or using them in skincare products or massage oils.

STARTING: APPLICATIONS FOR ESSENTIAL OILS

A thorough understanding of the range of essential oils and their various applications is necessary before beginning an aromatherapy journey. Essential oils can be grouped according to their therapeutic qualities, such as balancing, energizing, or calming. For instance, chamomile and bergamot oils are well-known for their calming effects, which encourage relaxation and stress relief, while peppermint and lemon oils are invigorating and can improve focus and mental clarity. Each oil's distinct aroma and qualities dictate its suitability for various purposes, such as enhancing immunity or encouraging sleep.

Aromatherapy can be experienced in several ways, such as inhalation, topical application, and diffusion. Diffusers are popular for dispersing essential oils into the air, creating a therapeutic atmosphere in homes or workplaces. Knowing these methods allows beginners to explore and integrate aromatherapy practices seamlessly into their daily lives, reaping the benefits of natural healing and well-being enhancement.

SAFETY POINTS TO REMEMBER

Aromatherapy has many advantages, but to guarantee a positive and safe experience, safety measures must be taken. Essential oils are strong substances that should be used carefully, particularly when applying directly to the skin or inhaling for long periods. Before using essential oils widely, it is best to conduct a patch test to rule out allergic reactions or sensitivities in certain individuals. Additionally, pregnant women, small children, and pets may be more sensitive to certain oils, so it is important to choose carefully and consult with healthcare professionals.

It is also necessary to follow recommended dilution ratios and usage guidelines provided by reliable sources or aromatherapy practitioners to preserve the potency and effectiveness of essential oils. It is important to educate oneself about the properties of each oil, as well as any potential interactions with medications and other relevant information to ensure responsible and effective use. By placing a high priority on safety precautions, people can confidently incorporate aromatherapy into their wellness routines, maximizing benefits while minimizing risks.

HOW YOU CAN BENEFIT FROM THIS BOOK

With a focus on safety to ensure that readers of all levels have a safe and enjoyable aromatherapy experience, this book serves as a comprehensive guide for those looking to explore the world of aromatherapy confidently and effectively. It covers essential topics such as understanding what aromatherapy is, its benefits across physical and emotional health, and practical advice on getting started with essential oils. Additionally, it offers detailed insights into selecting and using essential oils, exploring their diverse therapeutic properties and applications in daily life.

If you're new to aromatherapy, this book provides step-by-step instructions on how to incorporate essential oils into daily routines for relaxation, stress relief, or general well-being. It also offers helpful advice on selecting the appropriate oils, applying them, and blending them so that readers can tailor their practices to their own needs. Finally, the book answers common questions and concerns that beginners may have, such as how to store essential oils safely and how to get the most out of them.

CHAPTER TWO

COMPREHENDING AROMATHERAPY

THE ORIGINS AND HISTORY OF AROMATHERAPY

Thousands of years ago, aromatherapy was first used in ancient Egypt, Greece, and China, where people recognized the healing benefits of aromatic plants and their essential oils in treating a wide range of ailments and enhancing general well-being. In Egypt, aromatic oils were used in religious ceremonies and embalming practices, emphasizing their sacred and medicinal significance. Hippocrates and other Greek and Chinese medical figures further developed these practices, recording the medicinal benefits of aromatic substances for healing purposes. In Chinese traditional medicine, aromatic herbs and oils were incorporated into acupuncture and massage therapies to balance energy and treat illnesses.

Aromatherapy has developed over time in tandem with scientific understanding.

The term "aromatherapy" was first used in the 20th century by French chemist René-Maurice Gattefossé, who was inspired by the remarkable healing properties of lavender oil for burn patients. This discovery led to a systematic study of aromatherapy and its widespread use in holistic therapy and medical settings. Aromatherapy continues to combine traditional knowledge with modern science to provide natural remedies for physical, emotional, and mental well-being.

FUNDAMENTALS AND PRINCIPLES

Aromatherapy works on a few basic principles. Essential oils are concentrated compounds that are extracted from aromatic plants and interact with the body through inhalation, skin absorption, or ingestion (in some cases). Essential oils are known for their therapeutic properties, which can range from calming and uplifting effects to anti-microbial and anti-inflammatory effects. It is important to understand the purity and quality of essential oils;

reliable suppliers make sure the oils are derived from plants grown without pesticides and extracted using techniques that preserve their therapeutic potency.

Aromatherapy applies different application techniques based on the needs of each individual. Diffusers and direct palm inhalation allow oils to quickly enter the bloodstream through the lungs, affecting the nervous system and emotions. Topical application, diluted in carrier oils such as coconut or jojoba, targets specific areas for pain relief, skin improvement, or relaxation. Internal application, under professional guidance, involves ingesting oils for support of the digestive system or immune system. All application techniques follow safety guidelines, guaranteeing the safe and responsible use of essential oils.

ESSENTIAL OIL TYPES

Essential oils are a wide range of botanical extracts, each with specific therapeutic benefits. For example, peppermint oil, valued for its cooling effect, relieves headaches and digestive discomfort; tea tree oil, valued for its antibacterial and antifungal properties, treats skin conditions and strengthens immunity; citrus oils, such as lemon and orange, improve mood and focus, making them useful for fighting fatigue and fostering mental clarity; and eucalyptus oil, which clears sinuses and supports respiratory health, is useful during cold and flu seasons.

Selecting essential oils requires knowledge of each one's unique properties and intended application. Novices should begin with adaptable oils like peppermint and lavender and work their way up to more complex ones depending on their health objectives and preferences.

TECHNIQUES FOR EXTRACTING

The method used to extract essential oils determines their purity and therapeutic efficacy. The most popular method is steam distillation, which involves placing plant material in a distillation chamber and using steam to gently extract oils without compromising their chemical composition. Another method, known as solvent extraction, is less common but still effective for delicate flowers because it uses solvents to isolate the oils from plant materials. All of these methods produce different qualities and applications that guarantee versatility in aromatherapy practices.

Knowledge of extraction techniques enables practitioners to identify the qualities and uses of essential oils. Steam distillation retains the natural qualities of essential oils, making it appropriate for the majority of plant materials. Cold pressing preserves the vibrant, fruity scents of citrus oils, making them perfect for aromatherapy blends and household cleaning products.

ADVANTAGES NOT JUST IN SCENT

Beyond their pleasant scents, essential oils have many uses for holistic health. For example, diffusing lavender or chamomile oils promotes relaxation and lowers stress and anxiety levels.

Tea tree and eucalyptus oils are excellent topical treatments for skin infections and respiratory problems. Peppermint and rosemary oils, when applied topically, improve mental clarity and cognitive function. Finally, essential oils aid in detoxification, immune system support, and pain management, all of which contribute to general health and vitality.

Including essential oils in daily routines encourages emotional balance and natural healing. Essential oils have therapeutic effects that go beyond aroma; they influence physiological responses by directly interacting with the body's systems. Using oils in massage therapy, skincare routines, or diffuser blends improves wellness practices and offers natural substitutes for synthetic products. By utilizing the power of plant essences, people adopt holistic health approaches that are grounded in traditional wisdom as well as contemporary scientific validation.

CHAPTER THREE

OVERVIEW OF ESSENTIAL OILS

THE COMMON ESSENTIAL OILS AND THEIR CHARACTERISTICS

Essential oils are concentrated plant extracts with therapeutic benefits. Some of the most well-known oils are lavender, which is known for its ability to induce relaxation and aid in sleep; peppermint, which is valued for its stimulating aroma and capacity to reduce headaches and enhance concentration; and tea tree oil, which is well-known for its antiseptic qualities and efficacious treatment of fungal infections and acne. Each essential oil has distinct qualities derived from the plants from which it is extracted, such as eucalyptus, which is used for respiratory purposes, and lemon, which is known for its energizing qualities and immune-boosting qualities.

Understanding the unique qualities of each essential oil empowers users to choose the best ones for their needs, whether for aromatherapy, skincare, or household cleaning. For example, chamomile oil is valued for its soothing properties and is ideal for skin irritation and relaxation, while rosemary oil is favored for its stimulating effects and use in hair care. Quality varies significantly among brands, so look for oils that are pure, free of additives, and sourced from reputable suppliers to ensure potency and effectiveness.

When incorporating essential oils into daily routines, one way to do so is to dilute them with carrier oils such as jojoba or coconut oil before applying them topically or diffusing them into the air for aromatic benefits.

For example, cedarwood oil is highly valued for its grounding qualities and capacity to increase focus and relaxation, which makes it perfect for meditation or creating a peaceful atmosphere in homes. By learning about the properties of popular essential oils, beginners can effectively harness the benefits of these oils, which can promote well-being and improve the quality of daily life.

SELECTING HIGH-QUALITY OILS

Vetiver oil, with its grounding and balancing properties, is a prime example of the advantages of choosing oils sourced from sustainable practices that respect consumer health and the environment. When starting an essential oil journey, it is important to choose high-quality products to ensure safety and efficacy.

Quality oils are derived through careful extraction methods like steam distillation or cold pressing, preserving the plant's beneficial compounds without contamination. Look for oils labeled as 100% pure and organic, as these are less likely to contain synthetic additives or pesticides, ensuring a purer experience with potent therapeutic effects.

Understanding the importance of quality ensures that essential oils maintain their integrity and effectiveness over time, whether used for emotional support, respiratory health, or natural cleaning solutions. Lavender oil, for example, is cherished for its calming scent and versatile applications, from aiding sleep to soothing skin irritations. Assessing the oil's aroma, color, and consistency can provide clues to its purity and potency, with reputable brands offering detailed information on sourcing, testing, and certifications.

By prioritizing quality, beginners can confidently explore the diverse benefits of essential oils, promoting holistic well-being and enhancing everyday experiences with natural aromatics. For example, frankincense oil is revered for its spiritual and medicinal uses, making it a valuable addition to skincare regimens or meditation practices. Integrating quality essential oils into daily routines involves diluting them properly for topical use or diffusing them for aromatic benefits.

COMPREHENDING FRAGRANCE NOTES

Essential oils can be categorized into three main notes, each of which contributes unique characteristics to the overall aroma profile. Top notes, like citrus oils like bergamot or grapefruit, are light and uplifting, providing initial freshness and vitality. Middle notes, like geranium or lavender, offer floral or herbal scents that harmonize with both top and base notes, balancing the fragrance and adding depth. These scent notes are important concepts in creating harmonious and balanced blends for a variety of purposes.

Experimenting with scent notes allows beginners to explore the art of aromatherapy, tapping into the therapeutic potential of essential oils to enhance mood, alleviate stress, or promote physical well-being.

Base notes, such as sandalwood or patchouli, are rich and grounding, providing longevity to the scent blend and enhancing its overall stability.

Understanding these notes allows users to create personalized blends tailored to specific needs or preferences. For example, combining the earthy warmth of cedarwood with the floral sweetness of ylang-ylang can result in a calming blend perfect for relaxation or meditation.

Blending requires careful consideration of the volatility and aroma characteristics of the oils to make sure they work well together. For example, the grounding aroma of vetiver and the invigorating scent of peppermint oil combine to create a revitalizing blend that improves focus and clarity. By learning scent notes, beginners can blend essential oils with confidence to achieve desired effects, whether they are enhancing personal wellness routines or creating custom fragrances for natural home care products.

COMBINING FUNDAMENTALS

Understanding each essential oil's unique properties as well as how they work together to produce synergistic effects is the first step toward mastering the art of blending essential oils. Start by choosing oils that have complementary therapeutic benefits, like the uplifting qualities of lemon mixed with the calming influence of lavender. Experiment with different ratios to achieve desired scent profiles and therapeutic outcomes, adjusting concentrations based on personal preference and intended use. For example, blending eucalyptus with tea tree oil can produce a refreshing and purifying blend that's perfect for natural cleaning solutions or respiratory support.

If you are new to blending, you should take into account the viscosity and volatility of the oils as well as the intensity and longevity of the aroma. For example, combining a few drops of bergamot with a base note like cedarwood can result in a well-balanced blend that is appropriate for promoting relaxation or elevating mood. Using carrier oils such as almond or jojoba helps dilute strong essential oils while improving skin absorption and safety.

Finding distinctive blends that align with personal preferences and wellness objectives requires experimentation. For instance, blending geranium's floral notes with patchouli's earthy tones can produce a harmonious blend ideal for emotional balance or personal fragrance.

Recording blend recipes and tracking their results over time enables users to hone their blending abilities and effectively utilize the therapeutic potential of essential oils. By embracing the fundamentals of blending, novices can develop a deeper appreciation for aromatherapy and its life-changing benefits.

SHELF LIFE AND STORAGE

Lavender oil is a prime example of how important it is to store essential oils in cool, dark places to prolong shelf life and retain therapeutic benefits. Use airtight caps and keep bottles upright to minimize exposure to air and preserve the integrity of the oil. Essential oils should be stored in dark glass bottles away from direct sunlight and heat sources to prevent oxidation and degradation of their aromatic compounds.

To maintain quality and safety, users need to rotate their essential oils regularly and discard any that show signs of oxidation or have passed their expiration date. Users who are aware of the shelf life of essential oils can better manage their inventory and ensure that the oils remain potent for optimal use. Citrus oils, such as orange or lemon, have shorter shelf lives because of their higher volatility and susceptibility to oxidation.

Using essential oils in daily routines requires careful storage and using them within their recommended shelf life. For example, peppermint oil, which is prized for its cooling effect and support for the digestive system, needs to be stored properly to maintain its menthol content and aromatic freshness.

CHAPTER FOUR

BEGINNING AN AROMATHERAPY PRACTICE

ORGANIZING YOUR SPACE FOR AROMATHERAPY

Establishing a specific area for aromatherapy creates the ideal conditions for a restful and productive experience. Begin by selecting a peaceful location where you can decompress without disturbances. Ideally, this area should be well-ventilated and clutter-free to foster a tranquil atmosphere. Use natural light or soft lighting to promote relaxation. Set up cozy seating or cushions for your sessions. You can also incorporate calming decor or plants to add to the ambiance.

Next, arrange your supplies and essential oils in a way that makes sense to you. An aromatherapy box or tray can keep your oils organized and within easy reach. Label your oils so there is no confusion during sessions.

Add sensory-enhancing elements to your aromatherapy space, like soft music or ambient sounds, to further enhance the calming atmosphere. By carefully arranging your essential oils, you create a sanctuary where you can fully immerse yourself in the therapeutic benefits of essential oils.

ESSENTIAL INSTRUMENTS AND DEVICES

To effectively practice aromatherapy, assemble the necessary tools and equipment that will make your sessions easier. The foundation of aromatherapy is essential oils, so make sure to invest in high-quality oils from reliable suppliers. A diffuser is necessary to release aromatic molecules into the air; pick one that fits your needs and preferences, such as heat-based, nebulizing, or ultrasonic. Finally, be sure to stock up on carrier oils, such as sweet almond or jojoba, which dilute essential oils for safe topical application.

With the right tools on hand, you can effortlessly integrate aromatherapy into your daily routine and reap its therapeutic benefits.

Other helpful tools are glass droppers for accurate oil measurements, storage bottles to preserve custom blends, and inhalers for personal aromatherapy on the go. Make sure your tools are clean and well-maintained to preserve the integrity of your oils and blends.

SAFETY MEASURES

While using essential oils for aromatherapy, safety is of the utmost importance. Always dilute essential oils with a carrier oil before applying them to your skin to avoid irritation or sensitization. Before using essential oils widely, conduct a patch test on a small area of your skin to check for any adverse reactions. Keep essential oils out of the reach of pets and children as ingestion can be harmful. To keep essential oils potent, store them in dark, glass bottles out of direct sunlight.

You can safely and responsibly enjoy the therapeutic benefits of aromatherapy by following the manufacturer's instructions, never leaving a diffuser unattended, and avoiding prolonged exposure to concentrated essential oils in small, poorly ventilated spaces. If you have any health concerns or are pregnant, see a qualified aromatherapist or healthcare provider before using essential oils.

ESTABLISHING A CALM ENVIRONMENT

Setting up a calming environment is crucial to getting the most out of aromatherapy. Start by choosing essential oils that have a calming effect, like lavender, chamomile, or frankincense.

You can use these oils in massage blends or diffused to encourage relaxation and lower stress levels. Try different combinations of oils to find scents that speak to you personally.

Play calming music or enjoy the sounds of nature to further enhance relaxation. Think about adding elements like soft blankets or cushions to create a cozy and inviting space. Take time to breathe deeply and focus on the aromatic experience, allowing you to unwind and release tension. Through the use of soft lighting, such as candles or dimmable lamps, you can create a gentle ambiance.

USING AROMATHERAPY IN EVERYDAY SITUATIONS

By incorporating essential oils into your morning or evening routines, you can create custom blends for massage or skin care routines using oils known for their therapeutic properties.

You can also add a few drops of uplifting oils, like citrus or peppermint, to your shower or bath to invigorate your senses and improve overall well-being and balance.

Experience the benefits of aromatherapy on the go with a portable inhaler or diffuser necklace. Store essential oils near your desk or bed for easy access during the day. Try different application techniques, like topical application, inhalation, or aromatic baths, to find what works best for you.

By incorporating aromatherapy into your daily routine, you can take advantage of its potential to enhance mood, encourage relaxation, and support overall wellness.

CHAPTER FIVE

METHODS OF AROMATHERAPY

TECHNIQUES FOR INHALATION: STEAM INHALATION AND DIFFUSERS

One of the main ways to benefit from aromatherapy is through inhalation, which uses the power of essential oils in the air we breathe. Diffusers are common devices that distribute essential oils into the air, making it easy to inhale. They are available in different types, such as ultrasonic, nebulizing, and heat diffusers. Ultrasonic diffusers use water to distribute oils in a fine mist, which also helps to humidify the air. Nebulizing diffusers, on the other hand, break down oils into tiny particles without the need for water, which makes them perfect for concentrated aromatherapy. Heat diffusers use heat to evaporate oils, but they may change the chemical composition of delicate oils. Whichever diffuser you choose, make sure it is suitable for your needs and surroundings.

Another useful technique for inhaling is steam inhalation, which works especially well for sinus and respiratory problems. To practice steam inhalation, boil some water and pour it into a bowl. Then, add a few drops of essential oil, like peppermint or eucalyptus, to the hot water. Cover your head with a towel to form a tent over the bowl, then lean over it and breathe deeply for a few minutes. The aromatic molecules in the steam carry into your respiratory system, bringing relief and improving respiratory health. Remember to use hot water carefully to prevent burns, and make sure the space is well-ventilated.

TOPICAL USES: BATH AND MASSAGE BLENDS

Applying diluted essential oils topically to the skin allows for absorption and localized effects. Massage blends are popular because they combine the benefits of aromatherapy and physical touch therapy. To make a massage blend, dilute essential oils in a carrier oil such as jojoba or sweet almond oil.

For adults, the typical dilution ratio is 2-3 drops of essential oil per teaspoon of carrier oil, with sensitivity and age adjustments made. Blend oils that are known to be calming or energizing, like peppermint for a refreshing massage or lavender for relaxation. Apply the blend to the skin and massage lightly, allowing the oils to penetrate and benefit the skin and senses.

Aromatherapy can be enjoyed luxuriously with bath blends. To start, mix essential oils with a dispersant such as Epsom salts, milk, or carrier oil before adding them to the bathwater.

This will help the oils spread evenly in the water rather than float on the surface. Select oils that match your preferred type of bath, such as citrus oils for an energizing bath or lavender for relaxation. Then, soak in the bath for at least 15 to 20 minutes to maximize the therapeutic benefits of aromatherapy.

USING AROMATHERAPY IN SKINCARE

Essential oils are powerful plant extracts that have a variety of benefits, from anti-inflammatory to antioxidant. When incorporating essential oils into skincare routines, it's important to dilute them properly in a carrier oil that is suitable for your skin type. Jojoba oil, grapeseed oil, and coconut oil are popular choices as carriers because they work well with most skin types. For facial care, use lighter oils and lower concentrations—1-2 drops of essential oil per teaspoon of carrier oil—to avoid sensitizing delicate facial skin.

You can tailor your skincare routine by adding a few drops of essential oil to your moisturizer, facial serum, or facial mask. Before applying new oils, do a patch test to ensure compatibility and prevent allergic reactions. Over time, regular use of essential oils in skincare can promote clearer, healthier skin while offering the calming or uplifting effects of aromatherapy.

Choose essential oils known for their skincare benefits, such as tea tree oil for acne-prone skin, rosehip seed oil for anti-aging properties, or frankincense for rejuvenation.

BREATHING TO PROVIDE EMOTIONAL SUPPORT

Carrying a personal inhaler filled with a calming blend of oils like lavender, bergamot, and ylang-ylang can provide instant relief from stress and anxiety. Inhale deeply from the inhaler whenever you feel stressed or anxious, allowing the aromatic molecules to uplift your mood and promote relaxation. Aromatherapy inhalation techniques are widely used to support emotional well-being, offering natural remedies for stress, anxiety, and mood enhancement.

Aromatherapy inhalation can provide ongoing emotional support, helping you manage stress and maintain a positive mindset. Diffusers are excellent tools for continuous emotional support throughout the day.

Set up a diffuser in your home or workspace with oils known for their calming or uplifting properties. Essential oils like lavender, chamomile, and geranium can help reduce stress and anxiety levels while creating a soothing atmosphere. Experiment with different oil blends to find combinations that resonate with your emotions and preferences.

CLEANING USING ESSENTIAL OILS

Essential oils are flexible ingredients that can be used to create effective, non-toxic cleaning solutions. Because they are antibacterial, antiviral, and antifungal, they are perfect for disinfecting surfaces and leaving behind a pleasant aroma. To create an all-purpose cleaner, mix water, white vinegar, and essential oils in a spray bottle. For best results, choose cleansing and purifying oils like tea tree, lemon, or eucalyptus. Shake well before each use and spray onto surfaces before wiping with a cloth. This natural cleaner is safe for most surfaces, including countertops, sinks, and appliances.

Add a few drops of essential oil to a small jar or bowl of baking soda to create a revitalizing air freshener and deodorizer; place the open container in closets, bathrooms, or pet areas; the baking soda absorbs odors while the essential oils release aromatic molecules into the air, leaving behind a clean and fresh scent; you can even incorporate essential oils into your laundry routine by mixing them with unscented detergent or adding a few drops to dryer balls before beginning a load; this will not only give your clothes a natural scent, but it will also boost the antibacterial qualities of your laundry routine.

CHAPTER SIX
ADVANTAGES FOR WELLNESS AND HEALTH

RELAXATION AND STRESS REDUCTION

Aromatherapy is a widely accepted method of promoting relaxation and stress relief through the use of essential oils. Certain essential oils, such as lavender, chamomile, and frankincense, have calming effects on the nervous system when inhaled or applied topically. These oils can help reduce tension and anxiety by promoting the production of neurotransmitters like serotonin and dopamine, which are responsible for regulating mood and emotions. Including aromatherapy into your daily routine can create an environment that is soothing and encourages relaxation, making it a perfect activity for unwinding after a long day or during times of increased stress.

Aromatherapy is a great way to relieve stress. You can use a diffuser with a few drops of your favorite essential oil to fill the space with the aroma, or you can combine essential oils with a carrier oil like sweet almond or jojoba oil and apply the mixture to your wrists and temples for a calming effect all day long. Deep breathing the scent can intensify its calming effects and encourage calmness and relaxation. By adding aromatherapy into your self-care routine, you can effectively manage stress and cultivate a more balanced and peaceful mindset.

MOOD ELEVATION AND EMOTIONAL BALANCING

By stimulating the limbic system, the part of the brain that controls emotions and memories, essential oils like citrus (like bergamot and orange) and floral scents (like rose and geranium) can help improve mood and promote emotional stability. Aromatherapy is a powerful tool for balancing emotions through the therapeutic use of essential oils; it can reduce feelings of sadness or irritability and elevate mood.

Including aromatherapy in your daily routine can support emotional well-being by creating a positive and uplifting atmosphere.

To fully utilize the mood-boosting properties of aromatherapy, you should think about using a diffuser to spread your preferred essential oils throughout your home. You can also make your aromatherapy blend by combining a few drops of various oils and breathing in the aroma deeply. Using diluted essential oils topically can also help maintain a more balanced emotional state and enhance your general well-being.

ENHANCEMENT OF SLEEP

Incorporating aromatherapy into your evening routine can create a peaceful atmosphere that signals to your body that it's time to unwind and prepare for sleep. Certain essential oils, like lavender, cedarwood, and sandalwood, are renowned for their sedative properties, which can help calm the mind and prepare the body for restful sleep.

These oils work by influencing the production of neurotransmitters like serotonin and melatonin, which regulate sleep-wake cycles and promote deep relaxation.

Aromatherapy can help you sleep better. To start, diffuse your favorite essential oils in your bedroom about half an hour before bed. You can also add a few drops of essential oil to a warm bath or mix it with a carrier oil for a relaxing massage. Deeply inhaling the aroma and using relaxation techniques can also intensify the effects of aromatherapy on sleep. By incorporating aromatherapy into your nightly routine, you can create healthy sleep patterns and get more restorative sleep.

PAIN CONTROL

Essential oils such as peppermint, eucalyptus, and ginger have analgesic and anti-inflammatory properties that can relieve a variety of pains, such as headaches, muscle soreness, and stiff joints. These oils work by reducing inflammation, improving circulation, and blocking pain receptors in the body, providing targeted relief when applied topically or inhaled through aromatherapy practices. Including aromatherapy in your pain management strategy can complement other treatments and enhance overall well-being.

The best way to use aromatherapy for pain relief is to dilute the essential oils in a carrier oil and apply the mixture directly to the affected area, gently massaging it into the skin. You can also apply a few drops of essential oil to a hot or cold compress and apply it to the painful area for localized relief. Aromatherapy can also be used to improve your quality of life by reducing stress and promoting relaxation, which can further alleviate pain. You can use essential oils to treat pain locally and systemically by adding them to a hot or cold compress or diffuser.

INCREASING RESISTANT

Incorporating aromatherapy into your daily routine can support immune health and contribute to a stronger, more resilient body. Certain essential oils, such as tea tree, lemon, and eucalyptus, have antimicrobial, antiviral, and antifungal properties that can help strengthen the immune system and ward off infections. These oils work by supporting the body's natural defense mechanisms, such as stimulating white blood cell production and enhancing respiratory function, which can reduce the risk of illness and fast recovery from colds and flu.

Aromatherapy can be used to support immunity by diffusing immune-boosting essential oils in your home or place of business. You can also make your personal immunity blend by combining multiple oils and applying them to pulse points or the bottoms of your feet. Aromatherapy can be used to enhance the therapeutic effects and provide continuous immune support all day long. When used regularly as part of a holistic wellness approach, aromatherapy can support overall health and well-being and maintain optimal immune function.

CHAPTER SEVEN

AROMATHERAPY FOR PARTICULAR PURPOSES

AROMATHERAPY FOR DEPRESSION AND ANXIETY

Using the therapeutic properties of essential oils, aromatherapy provides a gentle yet effective way to manage anxiety and depression. Lavender oil is well known for its calming effects on the nervous system; its calming aroma helps reduce anxiety levels and promote relaxation.

You can use lavender oil for anxiety and depression by using an essential oil diffuser to diffuse it throughout your home or office, or you can dilute a few drops of lavender oil in a carrier oil like jojoba or sweet almond oil and apply it to your pulse points, like your wrists and temples, to apply the oil to your skin. This way, the oil is absorbed through the skin, offering continuous relief all day long.

Diffusing Bergamot oil in your home can create a refreshing and calming atmosphere. For topical application, mix a few drops of Bergamot oil with a carrier oil and massage it onto the skin. This can help alleviate feelings of sadness and promote a sense of well-being. Bergamot oil is another beneficial essential oil for anxiety and depression. Its citrusy and uplifting scent helps elevate mood and reduce stress levels.

Diffusing Frankincense oil during meditation or quiet times can help center the mind and reduce feelings of stress. You can also create a personal inhaler by adding a few drops of Frankincense oil onto a cotton ball or tissue and inhaling deeply whenever needed. This method provides quick relief and supports emotional stability throughout the day. Frankincense oil is also highly regarded for its grounding and balancing properties, which make it beneficial for managing emotions associated with anxiety and depression.

AROMATHERAPY FOR MIGRAINE AND HEADACHE RELIEF

Peppermint oil is well known for its analgesic properties, which help relax tense muscles and ease headache pain. To use peppermint oil for headaches, dilute a few drops in a carrier oil and apply it to your temples, forehead, and back of your neck.

This method provides a cooling sensation that can help soothe headaches effectively. Aromatherapy can be a natural remedy for headaches and migraines, offering relief without the side effects of medications.

Aside from diffusing the oil or inhaling straight from the bottle, eucalyptus is another effective essential oil for headaches because of its refreshing aroma, which can help clear nasal passages and reduce sinus pressure, which often contributes to headache discomfort. You can also blend eucalyptus oil with peppermint and lavender oils for a synergistic effect that targets both pain relief and relaxation.

Additionally, because of its analgesic and anti-inflammatory qualities, rosemary oil helps relieve tension headaches. A few drops of rosemary oil mixed with carrier oil, massaged into the forehead and temples, can help relieve headache symptoms. The stimulating aroma of rosemary oil also helps to improve circulation and mental clarity, which in turn helps to reduce the intensity of headaches.

ESSENTIAL OILS FOR DIGESTIVE HEALTH

Certain essential oils, such as ginger, which is known for its warming and soothing properties, can help alleviate nausea and improve digestion. You can dilute ginger oil in carrier oil and massage it onto your abdomen in a clockwise direction to stimulate digestion and relieve discomfort. Aromatherapy can support digestive health by easing symptoms such as bloating, indigestion, and nausea.

Diffusing Peppermint oil or inhaling it straight from the bottle can provide quick relief from indigestion.

You can also mix a few drops of Peppermint oil with a carrier oil and massage it onto your abdomen for soothing relief. Peppermint is another beneficial essential oil for digestive health because of its cooling sensation, which can help relax the muscles of the digestive tract, easing bloating and gas.

A drop or two of lemon oil added to a glass of water and consumed before meals can promote healthy digestion and reduce bloating. It can also aid in digestion by stimulating the production of gastric juices and enzymes. Moreover, lemon oil's fresh and citrusy aroma can help uplift mood while supporting digestive function.

AROMATHERAPY TO TREAT BREATHING PROBLEMS

Aromatherapy uses decongestant and expectorant essential oils to effectively treat respiratory conditions like congestion, coughs, and sinusitis. Eucalyptus oil is well known for its ability to unclog nasal passages and reduce respiratory discomfort;

you can diffuse it in your home or breathe it straight from the bottle to help clear your sinuses and facilitate easier breathing. You can also add a few drops of eucalyptus oil to hot water and inhale the steam to further open your airways.

Tea tree oil is another essential oil that is good for respiratory health. Its expectorant qualities help to clear mucus from the lungs, and its antimicrobial qualities help fight respiratory infections. You can diffuse tea tree oil in your bedroom or add it to a warm bath to help relieve coughs and congestion.

Due to its cooling and menthol properties, peppermint oil can also help relieve respiratory symptoms. You can apply peppermint oil to your chest and throat area for extra relief or you can inhale the oil straight from the bottle or diffuse it throughout the room to help clear your nasal congestion and encourage better breathing.

AROMATHERAPY TO HELP WITH CONCENTRATION AND FOCUS

Diffusing Rosemary oil in your workspace or inhaling it straight from the bottle can help sharpen focus and enhance memory retention. You can also blend Rosemary oil with Peppermint and Lemon oils for a revitalizing aroma that promotes sustained concentration.

Aromatherapy is a great way to use essential oils that stimulate the mind and improve cognitive function. Rosemary oil is well known for its ability to increase alertness and mental clarity.

Diffusing Lemon oil in the morning or during study sessions can promote a positive atmosphere for learning and productivity. You can also add a few drops of Lemon oil to a diffuser necklace or bracelet to enjoy its benefits on the go. Lemon is another effective essential oil for boosting focus. Its bright and citrusy scent can help uplift mood and improve mental agility.

Furthermore, by boosting alertness and decreasing mental fatigue, peppermint oil can support cognitive function. Its energizing aroma naturally boosts productivity throughout the day, and it can be applied topically to the temples and back of the neck to improve focus and clarity of thought.

CHAPTER EIGHT
HOMEMADE RECIPES FOR AROMATHERAPY
FUNDAMENTAL BLENDING METHODS

Learn the fundamentals of blending essential oils before beginning to work with DIY aromatherapy recipes. Choose your essential oils according to their therapeutic qualities and the scent profile you want. Popular choices include lavender for relaxation, peppermint for energy, and chamomile for calming effects. Use a carrier oil, such as sweet almond or jojoba oil, to dilute the potent essential oils and ensure safe application to the skin.

For best results, blend small amounts of oils in a clean glass bottle or bowl, adding drops of essential oils based on your recipe or preference (for example, 2 drops of lavender, 1 drop of cedarwood, and 1 drop of bergamot for a calming effect might be a typical blend). Note how many drops you use so that you can duplicate successful blends in the future.

Gently stir or swirl to thoroughly mix the oils without adding air bubbles.

Once blended, keep your aromatherapy oils in dark glass containers out of direct sunlight and heat to maintain their potency. Label each blend with its name and creation date for convenience. These fundamental blending methods serve as the basis for a variety of aromatherapy products that can be customized to meet your unique wellness needs and preferences, such as bath salts, room sprays, massage oils, and air fresheners.

CALM BATH SOAKS AND SALTS

After a long day, treat yourself to a relaxing bath or soak that will help you relax and rejuvenate. To begin, choose a base of Epsom or sea salts, which are well-known for their ability to relax and soothe muscles. In a mixing bowl, combine your chosen salts with carrier oil, like fractionated coconut oil, which helps distribute essential oils evenly in the bath water without leaving a greasy residue on the skin.

Then, add your chosen essential oils to the salt mixture. Lavender, chamomile, and ylang-ylang essential oils are good choices for a relaxing bath. Use ten to fifteen drops of essential oil per cup of salts, depending on your preferred scent and the strength of the oil. Stir the mixture well to ensure that the oils are evenly distributed throughout the salts.

After combining all the ingredients, pour your calming bath salts into pretty jars or airtight containers. Write the contents and suggested use (e.g., add a quarter to half a cup to warm bath water right before soaking) on the labels of each container. These homemade bath salts also make great gifts and customized candies.

RELAXING ROOM SPRAYS

Making relaxing room sprays lets you turn your living areas into peaceful retreats. To start, choose a base liquid, like witch hazel or distilled water, which serves as a vehicle for the essential oils. Then, fill a clean spray bottle with essential oils that are known to promote calm, like lavender, bergamot, and cedarwood.

Start with about 80–90ml of distilled water or witch hazel in a standard 100-spray bottle. Add 10–20 drops of essential oils, depending on your preferred level of fragrance intensity. Try different combinations until you get the scent profile you want. Before each use, gently shake the bottle to ensure the oils are evenly distributed.

Use your DIY room spray before meditation, yoga, or bedtime routines to enhance relaxation and reduce stress. These natural alternatives to commercial air fresheners are free of harmful chemicals and synthetic fragrances.

ENERGIZING OILS FOR MASSAGE

Energizing massage oils are ideal for reawakening fatigued muscles and stimulating the senses. Start by choosing carrier oil, like sweet almond oil or grapeseed oil, which absorbs easily into the skin and supplies vital nutrients. Next, mix your selected carrier oil with energizing essential oils, like eucalyptus and peppermint, as well as citrus oils, like lemon or orange.

Use about 20 drops of essential oil per 30ml of carrier oil for a calming yet invigorating massage blend; adjust the ratio according to your preferred level of scent intensity and the purpose of the massage oil. Tightly seal the bottle and gently shake to completely blend the oils before each use, making sure the essential oils are evenly distributed throughout the carrier oil.

Enjoy the revitalizing effects of this DIY aromatherapy product as part of your self-care routine. Apply your invigorating massage oil to clean, dry skin using gentle, circular motions. Concentrate on areas of tension or fatigue, such as the neck, shoulders, and back, to promote relaxation and relieve muscle soreness. Store your massage oil in a cool, dark place between uses to maintain its freshness and potency.

ALL-NATURAL AIR FRESHENERS

You can enjoy pleasant scents throughout your home without using synthetic chemicals by making your natural air fresheners. First, choose a base (baking soda or vodka works well for this), and then mix your chosen essential oils (like lemon, tea tree, and lavender) with your chosen base in a small bowl.

If you want to use vodka as the base, mix 1/4 cup of vodka with 20–30 drops of essential oils in a spray bottle and shake well before each use to blend the ingredients. Alternatively, for a more straightforward but effective air freshener, mix about 1/2 cup of baking soda with 20–30 drops of essential oils. Stir the mixture well to distribute the oils throughout the baking soda.

These DIY air fresheners are affordable, customizable, and eco-friendly, providing a healthier substitute for commercial air freshener products.

CHAPTER NINE

INCLUDING AROMATHERAPY IN EVERYDAY ACTIVITIES

AROMATHERAPY IN WORKPLACES AND OFFICES

Aromatherapy diffusers are a great way to introduce aromatherapy into your office space and improve both productivity and well-being. To start, choose essential oils that have a calming or invigorating effect, like lavender for relaxation or peppermint for focus. You can also make your inhaler by adding a few drops of oil to a cotton pad or tissue for on-the-go relief.

A designated relaxation space can be created by setting up a calming corner with a diffuser or oil burner. Aromatherapy can also be applied topically using diluted oils for massage during breaks, promoting stress relief and muscle relaxation. It is important to take into account your coworkers' sensitivities and preferences when incorporating aromatherapy into your workspace. Additionally, opt for milder scents that aren't overpowering, and make sure there is adequate ventilation.

Making aromatherapy a daily routine at work can help you focus better, manage stress, and create a more pleasant and productive environment. Try experimenting with different oil combinations to find combinations that work best for your team. Aromatherapy can be incorporated into office culture to foster a more positive atmosphere and improve overall morale.

USING AROMATHERAPY IN MEDITATION AND YOGA

Essential oils that support your goals (e.g., lavender for relaxation, frankincense for spiritual connection, or eucalyptus for clarity) can be used to deepen the benefits of yoga and meditation practices by improving relaxation and concentration. Diffusers work great in yoga studios, dispersing oils into the air to create a calming atmosphere.

You can also apply diluted oils directly to pulse points or use them in massage oils for even more profound relaxation.

Aromatherapy can help clear the mind and create a peaceful atmosphere during meditation. You can incorporate essential oils into your pre-meditation routines by diffusing them in your meditation space or dabbing a few drops onto a tissue that is placed nearby.

This practice can help you focus and experience mindfulness more fully. When you practice yoga, essential oils can improve your breathing exercises and encourage relaxation in general.

You can reap the benefits of aromatherapy even after your session by diffusing oils in your space or using them topically for ongoing relaxation. When you incorporate aromatherapy into your yoga and meditation practices, you can create a more fulfilling and immersive experience that improves your mental and emotional well-being.

USING AROMATHERAPY WHILE TRAVELING

Choose travel-friendly essential oils like peppermint for energy, chamomile for calming, or citrus oils for a refreshing pick-me-up. Portable diffusers or personal inhalers are convenient ways to enjoy aromatherapy during travel—simply add a few drops of oil and inhale deeply for instant relief. Aromatherapy can be a soothing companion during travel, helping to ease stress and promote relaxation on the go.

Aromatherapy can help reduce anxiety and fatigue associated with travel. It can also help combat jet lag by promoting restful sleep and helping you adjust to new time zones.

Use an aroma stick or travel-sized diffuser to create a relaxing atmosphere in your hotel room or cabin. You can also apply diluted oils to pulse points or use them in massage oils to relax muscles and ease tension.

Packing a small kit of essential oils and travel accessories will allow you to incorporate aromatherapy into your routine. Try different oil combinations to find what works best for your needs and preferences. Whenever you travel, you can improve your relaxation, lower your stress level, and have a more comfortable trip.

AROMATHERAPY USES ON PETS

Aromatherapy is a great way to help your pets relax, reduce anxiety, and support overall well-being. However, before using essential oils, make sure they are safe for your particular pet species—dogs, cats, and other animals may have different sensitivities. Choose essential oils that are safe for pets, like lavender, which is calming, chamomile, which is grounding, and cedarwood, which is relaxing. You should always dilute essential oils with a carrier oil before applying them to prevent skin irritation.

Aromatherapy can be applied to pets through diffusion in a well-ventilated area or by diluting oils to bedding or collars; start with small amounts and watch your pet's reactions to make sure they are comfortable with the scent; unless instructed by a veterinarian, avoid applying directly to pets' fur or skin.

Aromatherapy can also be used to soothe and support your pet during stressful events like vet visits or travel.

Using aromatherapy as part of a holistic approach to pet care, along with regular veterinary check-ups and a balanced diet, can improve your pet's quality of life and strengthen your bond with them. Gradually introduce aromatherapy into your pet's routine, keeping an eye on their reaction and making adjustments as necessary.

CHILDREN AND FAMILIES WITH AROMATHERAPY

Use child-friendly essential oils like lavender for relaxation, chamomile for soothing, or citrus oils for uplifting spirits. Always dilute essential oils appropriately before use, especially for children, to prevent skin sensitivity or adverse reactions.

Use diffusers or aroma sticks in common areas of the home to create a comforting ambiance. Aromatherapy can be a gentle and effective way to support children's well-being and promote a calm, nurturing environment at home.

Aromatherapy can be used during playtime or study sessions to enhance focus and concentration. For family gatherings or special occasions, create a welcoming atmosphere by diffusing festive essential oil blends. F

or children, aromatherapy can be integrated into bedtime routines to promote relaxation and support restful sleep. Add a few drops of calming oils to a bedtime bath or diffuse oils in their bedroom before bedtime.

Embrace aromatherapy into your family's daily routine by getting the kids involved in choosing and applying scents, making sure they feel at ease and involved, and keeping an eye on how they react to various oils so you can make adjustments based on their preferences and sensitivities. Aromatherapy can help your family feel better overall, feel less stressed, and foster a loving environment that everyone can enjoy.

CHAPTER TEN
SAFETY AND PRECAUTIONS
GUIDELINES FOR ESSENTIAL OIL DILUTION

A general rule of thumb is to dilute essential oils before applying them topically. The recommended dilution ratio varies depending on factors like the specific oil, the intended use, and the individual's sensitivity. For topical application, adults should typically dilution at a ratio of 2-3 drops of essential oil per teaspoon (5 mL) of carrier oil; for children or those with sensitive skin, a lower dilution ratio is recommended, typically 1 drop of essential oil per teaspoon of carrier oil. Understanding proper dilution is crucial when using essential oils for aromatherapy. Essential oils are highly concentrated extracts derived from plants, and using them undiluted can cause skin irritation or other adverse reactions.

Before using diluted essential oils on a larger area of the skin, it is imperative to conduct a patch test to ascertain whether any sensitivity or allergic reaction is present. To do this, dilute the essential oil as directed, apply a small amount to a patch of skin (e.g., the inner forearm), and observe any adverse reactions for 24 hours. If irritation occurs, stop using the oil immediately and wash the area with mild soap and water. Diluted essential oils should always be stored in dark glass bottles to preserve their potency and avoid degradation.

ALLERGIES AND SENSITIVITIES

When using aromatherapy with essential oils, it is important to understand sensitivities and allergies. Although essential oils have many therapeutic benefits, some people may experience allergic reactions or sensitivities to them. Common signs of sensitivity or allergy include skin irritation, redness, itching, or respiratory problems like congestion or sneezing. Because of their chemical makeup, some essential oils, like peppermint or citrus oils, are more likely to cause sensitivities.

If you have known allergies to particular plants or substances, check the botanical source of the essential oil to avoid potential allergens. When diffusing essential oils, ensure proper ventilation and avoid prolonged exposure in enclosed spaces, especially for individuals with respiratory conditions or sensitivities.

When applying essential oils topically or in a diffuser, always dilute them properly before use. Consider conducting a patch test before full application to assess individual sensitivity.

AROMATHERAPY AND PREGNANCY

Due to the potential effects on the developing fetus as well as the mother, aromatherapy during pregnancy presents special considerations. Certain essential oils, like clary sage or basil, are known to stimulate menstruation or contractions and should be avoided completely, but others are generally considered safe when used in moderation and with appropriate dilution.

See a qualified healthcare professional, such as an obstetrician or midwife, before using essential oils during pregnancy to ensure safety. Certain essential oils can alter hormone levels or circulation, which may have an impact on the course of the pregnancy. Use low concentrations of mild, calming essential oils, such as lavender or chamomile, and avoid ingesting essential oils during pregnancy as this can carry significant risks. If you are unsure about a particular essential oil, err on the side of caution and wait to use it until after pregnancy and breastfeeding.

INTERACTIONS BETWEEN DRUGS

Essential oils contain bioactive compounds that may interact with prescription drugs, over-the-counter medications, or supplements. Citrus oils, such as grapefruit oil, can interfere with liver enzymes that metabolize medications, resulting in either increased or decreased drug levels in the bloodstream. It is important to understand potential interactions between essential oils and medications because some oils can affect how medications are metabolized or their effectiveness.

Consider using essential oils in ways that minimize systemic absorption, such as inhalation or diluted topical application. If experiencing any unexpected side effects while using essential oils with medications, discontinue use and seek medical advice promptly. Before using essential oils alongside medications, consult with a healthcare professional, such as a pharmacist or physician, to review potential interactions. Inform them of all medications and supplements you are currently taking to ensure compatibility with essential oils.

TIPS FOR SAFE HANDLING AND STORAGE

Essential oils should always be kept out of the reach of children and pets to prevent accidental ingestion or spills. Proper handling and storage are crucial to preserving the potency of essential oils and ensuring safety.

Essential oils should be stored in dark glass bottles in a cool, dry place away from sunlight and heat sources.

Wear gloves or a dropper when handling undiluted essential oils, and make sure you have enough ventilation when diffusing them to prevent respiratory irritation. Dispose of expired or oxidized essential oils properly by local regulations to minimize environmental impact. Exercise caution when handling essential oils, especially undiluted oils, to avoid direct contact with the skin. If accidental skin contact occurs, wash the affected area immediately with soap and water to dilute the oil and prevent irritation.

Understanding these important factors—dilution, sensitivities, pregnancy considerations, medication interactions, and proper handling—lays a solid foundation for a safe and enjoyable aromatherapy experience. By adhering to these recommendations, people can responsibly and confidently harness the therapeutic potential of essential oils.

CHAPTER ELEVEN

FAQS & FREQUENTLY ASKED QUESTIONS

DISPELLING MYTHS ABOUT ESSENTIAL OILS

There are a few common misconceptions about essential oils that can make it difficult for newcomers to understand them. Firstly, there is a common misconception that essential oils can treat serious medical conditions on their own. It is important to clarify that although essential oils have therapeutic benefits, they should not be used in place of medical treatment for conditions like diabetes or cancer. Secondly, there is a misconception about the safety of ingesting essential oils. You should always seek the advice of a qualified aromatherapist before ingesting any essential oils. Lastly, it is important to dispel the myth that all essential oils are safe to use; some oils can cause allergic reactions or skin sensitivities, which highlights the significance of patch testing.

Beginners must prioritize pure, high-quality essential oils to maximize therapeutic benefits and avoid potential risks associated with synthetic alternatives. Pure essential oils are derived from natural plant sources through processes like distillation, ensuring they retain therapeutic properties. On the other hand, fragrance oils are synthetic and lack the same therapeutic benefits.

While there are many different brands of essential oils, novices should focus on trustworthy businesses that have a reputation for openness and quality control. Finding out about a company's sourcing policies, testing procedures, and customer feedback can reveal important information about how reliable their products are. Look for brands that offer comprehensive details about the botanical species used, extraction techniques, and any third-party testing for purity and potency. While quality oils may seem more costly upfront, they will pay off in the long run by providing safer and more effective aromatherapy experiences.

AROMATHERAPY IN COMBINATION WITH OTHER THERAPIES

Combining aromatherapy with other therapeutic practices can improve overall effectiveness and well-being. For example, diffusing relaxing oils like lavender during meditation sessions can deepen relaxation and promote mental clarity, enhancing the benefits of mindfulness practices. Another potent combination is blending aromatherapy with massage therapy. Essential oils can complement massage techniques by promoting relaxation, easing muscle tension, and enhancing the overall therapeutic experience.

If you're interested in incorporating aromatherapy into your skincare routine, you can safely apply essential oils topically by diluting them in carrier oils like jojoba or coconut oil. Depending on your skin type and desired results, you may want to try tea tree oil for acne-prone skin or rose oil for anti-aging benefits. However, be careful when diluting essential oils to prevent irritation of your skin, especially on delicate areas like your face or neck.

Whether utilizing aromatherapy for mood enhancement, skincare, or relaxation, integrating it with other therapeutic practices can amplify its benefits and create a more holistic approach to wellness. Individual preferences and sensitivities should be taken into consideration when combining aromatherapy with other therapies. Some people may find certain essential oil blends more enjoyable or effective than others, so experimentation and personalization are key.

SELECTING REPUTABLE BRANDS OF ESSENTIAL OILS

When it comes to ensuring safety and efficacy in aromatherapy practices, choosing high-quality brands of essential oils is crucial. Start your research by looking for brands that place a high value on transparency and follow stringent quality standards in both production and sourcing.

Reputable brands frequently offer comprehensive information about their sourcing practices, including the specific botanical species used, cultivation techniques, and extraction processes. Look for brands that carry out independent testing to confirm the purity and potency of their oils, guaranteeing they are free from contaminants and adulterants.

A brand's overall satisfaction and dependability can be determined by looking at customer reviews and feedback. Good reviews typically point to consistent product quality and customer service, while bad reviews can draw attention to problems like packaging leaks or inconsistent scent profiles. You should also look for brands that provide instructional materials and advice on safe usage procedures, such as dilution ratios and possible contraindications.

A beginner should prioritize buying essential oils from reliable suppliers or retailers that specialize in aromatherapy products to ensure they receive genuine and effective oils for their wellness needs.

Price can also play a role in the selection of essential oils, as higher-quality oils often come with a higher price tag. However, investing in reputable brands known for their purity and therapeutic benefits can provide greater value and safety in the long run.

PROBLEM-SOLVING CHALLENGES

Achieving the desired scent intensity when diffusing essential oils is a common challenge, but knowing how to troubleshoot and address it can improve the overall experience. Changing the number of drops used or experimenting with different oil combinations can help achieve the desired aroma strength without overwhelming the senses. Cleaning the diffuser regularly and using distilled water can prevent clogging and ensure optimal diffusion efficiency.

Patch testing a small area of skin before widely using essential oils can help identify any potential allergic reactions or sensitivities, ensuring safe and comfortable aromatherapy experiences.

Skin sensitivity or irritation from essential oils is another problem that beginners may encounter, especially when applying them topically. Diluting essential oils in a carrier oil like almond or grapeseed oil can reduce the risk of irritation and enhance absorption into the skin.

Consistency in aromatherapy practices is key to optimizing therapeutic benefits. Essential oils should be stored in a cool, dark place away from heat and direct sunlight to maintain their potency and shelf life. Properly closing bottles after each use and using amber or dark-colored glass containers can further prevent oils from deteriorating. Novices can improve their aromatherapy experiences and reap the benefits of essential oils by following best practices and troubleshooting common issues.

LOCATING TRUSTED SOURCES

The National Association for Holistic Aromatherapy (NAHA) and the Alliance of International Aromatherapists (AIA) are two reputable organizations that offer valuable educational resources, including articles, webinars, and certification programs that promote safe usage practices and deepen understanding of aromatherapy principles. While navigating the vast array of aromatherapy resources can be daunting for beginners, finding reliable sources is crucial for safe and effective practice.

Online communities and forums devoted to aromatherapy can also be invaluable resources for exchanging experiences, asking questions, and gaining knowledge from others' insights and expertise. Books written by certified aromatherapists and reputable experts can also offer comprehensive guidance on essential oil profiles, therapeutic uses, and blending techniques. Look for books that cite scientific research and include useful applications for everyday use, ensuring the information is both accurate and accessible.

A beginner can confidently incorporate essential oils into their wellness routines by accessing reliable online resources and staying informed. When consulted online, prioritize websites and blogs run by qualified aromatherapists or accredited institutions. Verify the credentials and expertise of authors to ensure the information presented is credible and evidence-based. Avoid sources that make exaggerated claims or promote unsafe practices, as misinformation can lead to improper use of essential oils and potential health risks.

www.ingramcontent.com/pod-product-compliance
Lightning Source LLC
Chambersburg PA
CBHW061253250726

48653CB00002B/637